ILLUSTRATED GUIDE TO MALFORMATIONS OF THE CENTRAL NERVOUS SYSTEM AT BIRTH

GUIDE ILLUSTRÉ DES MALFORMATIONS DU SYSTÈME NERVEUX CENTRAL À LA NAISSANCE

ILLUSTRIERTER LEITFADEN DER MIßBILDUNGEN DES ZENTRALNERVENSYSTEMS BEI DER GEBURT

COMMISSION OF THE EUROPEAN COMMUNITIES

ILLUSTRATED GUIDE TO MALFORMATIONS OF THE CENTRAL NERVOUS SYSTEM AT BIRTH

GUIDE ILLUSTRÉ DES MALFORMATIONS DU SYSTÈME NERVEUX CENTRAL À LA NAISSANCE

ILLUSTRIERTER LEITFADEN DER MIßBILDUNGEN DES ZENTRALNERVEN-SYSTEMS BEI DER GEBURT

Norman C. Nevin

MD BSc FRCP Ed FRCPath FFCM
Professor of Medical Genetics, Queen's University of Belfast

Josephine A.C. Weatherall

MB ChB BSc FFCM
Project Leader, EUROCAT:
Registration of Congenital Abnormalities and Twins

Churchill Livingstone ▦
EDINBURGH LONDON MELBOURNE AND NEW YORK 1983

Published for the
Commission of the European Communities,
Directorate-General Information Market and Innovation,
Luxembourg

EUR 7074

Contract No. 1-78-1 MRB

EUROCAT Central Registry
EPID 30.34—Clos Chapelle Aux Champs 30, B-1200 Bruxelles

LEGAL NOTICE
Neither the Commission of the European Communities nor any person acting on behalf
of the Commission is responsible for the use which might be made of the following
information

Cataloguing data can be found at the end of this publication

©ECSC-EEC-EAEC, Brussels and Luxembourg, 1983

ISBN 0 443 02635 1 (Churchill Livingstone)
ISBN 3 432 93191 3 (Enke) .

Printed in Hong Kong by C & C Joint Printing Co., (H.K.) Ltd.

This book has been prepared in order to allow relatively inexperienced doctors, midwives and pathologists to make correct diagnoses of babies born with visible congenital malformations of the central nervous system. There is a foreword and a brief description of how to examine a newborn infant. This is followed by descriptions, photographs in colour and line drawings of 12 of the 13 major congenital malformations of the central nervous system including anencephalus, iniencephalus, spina bifida, cranial meningocele, hydrocephaly, arhinencephaly and microcephaly. An appendix includes a classification of the central nervous system malformations along with variants and many synonymous terms.

Foreword

Preface

Vorwort

This book has been produced as one of the outcomes of a workshop on the recording of central nervous system malformations held in Brussels in December 1979 as part of the EUROCAT coordination programme.

EUROCAT is the acronym for the EEC concerted Action Project—Registration of Congenital Abnormalities and Twins which was started in 1978. The objective is to establish within defined geographic areas, the registration of all babies born, alive or dead, which are of multiple births or which have a congenital abnormality of a structural or functional nature and whose mother is resident in the defined geographic area. The methods for reporting cases to the EUROCAT centre are now established and research into the clarification and the standardisation of diagnosis and nomenclature for different groups of malformation is part of the EUROCAT project. The registries so created will form reference centres for further epidemiological and preventive studies.*

The workshop on the recording of central nervous system malformations was the first of the attempts to standardise diagnosis. The following consultants assisted in the workshop:

> *Professor Verne S. Caviness*, Eunice Kennedy Schriver Centre for Mental Retardation, INC, Massachusetts, USA
> *Professor F. Evrard*, Clinique St Luc, Catholic University of Louvain, Brussels, Belgium

Ce livre est issu des travaux d'un séminaire consacré à l'enregistrement des malformations congénitales du système nerveux central qui s'est tenu à Bruxelles en décembre 1979 dans le cadre de la coordination du programme EUROCAT.

EUROCAT est le sigle du Projet d'Action Concertée de la Communauté Economique Européenne pour l'Enregistrement des Anomalies Congénitales et des Naissances Multiples—Projet qui débuta en 1978 et dont l'objectif est d'établir dans des zones géographiques définies, un système d'enregistrement des naissances multiples ainsi que de tout enfant né-vivant ou mort-né qui présente une anomalie congénitale de structure ou de fonction et dont la mère réside dans la zone géographique définie. Actuellement, les procédures de notification des cas au Centre Coordinateur EUROCAT sont établies, cependant que les recherches se poursuivent pour clarifier et standardiser le diagnostic et la nomenclature des différents groupes de malformations. Les zones où les registres sont ainsi crées serviront de centre de référence pour des futures études épidémiologiques et de prévention.*

Le séminaire sur l'enregistrement des malformations du système nerveux central est la première tentative de standardisation des diagnostics. Les personnes suivantes y ont assisté:

> *Professor Verne S. Caviness*, Eunice Kennedy Schriver Centre for Mental Retardation, INC,

Dieses Buch verdankt seine Entstehung der Tagung einer Arbeitsgruppe, die sich im Dezember 1979 in Brüssel mit der Registrierung von Mißbildungen des Zentralnervensystems als Teilprojekt des EUROCAT-Koordinationsprogramms befaßte.

EUROCAT ist das Kurzwort für das 1978 begonnene Aktionsprojekt im Rahmen der EG zur Registrierung von angeborenen Anomalien und von Zwillingen. Endziel soll die Erfassung und die Registrierung, in geographisch begrenzten Gebieten, aller Säuglinge sein, die lebend oder tot, als Mehrfachgeburt oder mit einer angeborenen strukturell oder funktionell bedingten Anomalie zur Welt kommen und deren Mütter in den besagten geographisch begrenzten Gebieten leben. Die Modalitäten zur Anmeldung der Fälle bei den EUROCAT-Zentralstellen sind schon festgelegt worden; das EUROCAT-Projekt befaßt sich jetzt u.a. mit der Klärung und Vereinheitlichung der Diagnosen und der Terminologie für verschiedene Mißbildungsgruppen. Die auf diese Weise entstandenen Register werden Referenzzentren für weitere epidemiologische und Vorsorge-Studien werden.*

Die Bildung der Arbeitsgruppe für die Registrierung von Mißbildungen des Zentralnervensystems war der erste Versuch, die Diagnosen zu vereinheitlichen. Folgende fachärztliche Berater halfen dabei:

> *Professor Verne S. Caviness*, Eunice Kennedy Schriver Centre

---

*A list of registries is included in Appendix II.

*La liste des Centres est présentée en annexe II.

*Eine Liste der Register ist im Anhang II beigefügt.

Dr Angus Gibson, Royal Hospital for Sick Children, University of Glasgow, UK
Professor F. Gullotta, University of Bonn, West Germany
Mr L.P. Lassman, Royal Victoria Hospital, Newcastle upon Tyne, UK
Professor K.M. Laurence, Welsh National School of Medicine, University of Wales, UK
Professor G. Lyon, Clinique St Luc, Catholic University of Louvain, Brussels, Belgium
Dr Pierpaolo Mastroiacovo, Catholic University of Rome, Italy
Professor Norman C. Nevin, The Queen's University of Belfast, UK
Professor Charles Roux, Hospital St Antoine, University of Paris, France

The basis of discussion was the classification of central nervous system defects currently presented in the Ninth Revision of the International Classification of Disease (ICD). Using this, and the terms included in the index to the Ninth Revision of the ICD, a modified classification was prepared which was accepted unanimously. This classification is shown in Appendix I; its inclusion in this book is to help clarify the jungle of diagnostic terms which are at present being used in clinical work in connection with infants who have central nervous system malformations.

The book has been kept simple to permit easy and quick reference and to allow correct diagnosis to be reached by relatively unskilled medical personnel.

Massachusetts, USA
Professeur P. Evrard, Clinique St Luc, Université Catholique de Louvain, Bruxelles, Belgique
Dr Angus Gibson, Royal Hospital for Sick Children, University of Glasgow, UK
Professor F. Gullotta, University of Bonn, West Germany
Mr L.P. Lassman, Royal Victoria Hospital, Newcastle upon Tyne, UK
Professor K.M. Laurence, Welsh National School of Medicine, University of Wales, UK
Professeur G. Lyon, Clinique St Luc, Université Catholique de Louvain, Bruxelles, Belgique
Dr Pierpaolo Mastroiacovo, Université Catholique de Rome, Italie
Professor Norman C. Nevin, The Queen's University of Belfast, UK
Professeur Charles Roux, Hôpital St Antoine, Université de Paris, France

La classification des anomalies du système nerveux central telle que présentée dans la neuvième Révision de la classification internationale des Maladies (C.I.M.) a servi de base à la discussion. Utilisant cette classification ainsi que les termes repris dans l'index de la neuvième Révision de la C.I.M., une classification modifiée a été élaborée et acceptée à l'unanimité par les participants. Cette classification est présentée en annexe I. Son inclusion dans ce livre a pour but de clarifier la terminologie à présent utilisée dans les travaux cliniques relatifs aux anomalies du système nerveux central.

Ce livre se veut élémentaire afin

for Mental Retardation, INC., Massachusetts, USA
Professor F. Evrard, Clinique St. Luc, Catholic University of Louvain, Brussels, Belgium
Dr Angus Gibson, Royal Hospital for Sick Children, University of Glasgow, UK
Professor F. Gullotta, Institut für Neuropathologie, Universität Bonn, BRO
Mr L.P. Lassman, Royal Victoria Hospital, Newcastle upon Tyne, UK
Professor K.M. Laurence, Welsh National School of Medicine, University of Wales, UK
Professor G. Lyon, Clinique St Luc, Catholic University of Louvain, Brussels, Belgium
Dr Pierpaolo Mastroiacovo, Catholic University of Rome, Italy
Professor Norman C. Nevin, The Queen's University of Belfast, UK
Professor Charles Roux, Hôpital St Antoine, University of Paris, France

Als Diskussionsgrundlage diente die Klassifikation der zentralnervösen Mißbildungen, wie sie derzeit in der neunten Auflage der International Classification of Diseases (ICD) vorliegt. Anhand dieser und unter Einbeziehung der in dem Index zur neunten Auflage erwähnten Bezeichnungen wurde eine modifizierte Klassifikation ausgearbeitet, die einstimmig angenommen wurde. Diese Klassifikation zeigt Anhang I; ihre Integrierung in dieses Buch soll dazu beitragen, die Überzahl von diagnostischen Bezeichnungen, die zur Zeit— um Mißbildungen des Zentral-

de fournir une référence simple et
rapide et de permettre à des personnes non spécialisées de poser
un diagnostic correct.

nervensystems bei Säuglingen zu
beschreiben—in der klinischen
Praxis in Gebrauch sind, auf ein
Minimum zu reduzieren.

Der Inhalt dieses Buches wurde
bewußt einfach gehalten und soll es
dem relativ ungeschulten Personal
ermöglichen, rasch nachzuschlagen
und die richtige Diagnose zu
stellen.

Contents

Sommaire

Inhaltsverzeichnis

Recognition of central nervous system malformations

Malformations of the central nervous system (CNS) are among the most frequent and the most tragic of congenital disorders which afflict man. The incidence at birth of some CNS malformations, such as anencephalus and spina bifida, show considerable geographic variation both between and within countries. In the United Kingdom, high rates are found in Northern Ireland and Scotland, whereas in Japan the frequency is low. Recognition of specific CNS malformations is important particularly in epidemiological studies. There is an increasing awareness of the aetiologic heterogeneity of some CNS malformations. In terms of aetiology the major part of anencephalus and spina bifida has probably a multifactorial origin. Some, for example in Meckel's syndrome or in Robert's syndrome, are due to major genes. Others, although rarely, may be associated with a chromosomal abnormality. Accurate diagnosis is important in the prevention of CNS malformations through genetic counselling and prenatal diagnosis. The aim of this book is to provide to medical personnel concerned with the newborn a ready reference to the recognition of some of the most common CNS malformations.

Identification des malformations du système nerveux central

Les malformations du système nerveux central (SNC) sont au nombre des anomalies congénitales les plus fréquentes et les plus sévères. La fréquence à la naissance de certaines malformations comme l'anencéphalie et le spina bifida indique des variations géographiques importantes aussi bien entre pays qu'au sein d'un même pays. Au Royaume-Unis, on observe des taux élevés en Irlande du Nord et en Ecosse, alors qu'au Japon, les taux sont faibles. L'identification des malformations spécifiques du SNC est importante, particulièrement pour les études épidémiologiques. L'étiologie des malformations du SNC est semble-t-il, des plus hétérogène. La plupart des anencéphalies et spina bifida ont probablement une étiologie multifactorielle. Le syndrome de Meckel ou le syndrome de Robert sont dus à des anomalies génomiques. D'autre malformations rares sont associées à des anomalies chromosomiques. Un diagnostic précis des malformations du SNC est important pour évaluer l'intérêt de l'impact d'une prévention par le conseil génétique ou le diagnostic pré-natal. L'objectif de ce livre est de fournir au personnel médical et para-médical une référence pour le diagnostic des malformations du SNC les plus courantes.

Zur Erkennung von Mißbildungen des Zentralnervensystems

Mißbildungen des Zentralnervensystems (ZNS) gehören zu den häufigsten angeborenen Störungen, die den Menschen heimsuchen. Das Vorkommen einiger solcher Mißbildungen, wie z.B. Anenzephalie oder Spina bifida, zeigen merkwürdige geographische Abweichungen zwischen einzelnen Ländern, aber auch innerhalb eines und desselben Landes. In Großbritannien z.B. sind die Mißbildungsraten besonders hoch in Nordirland und Schottland, während in Japan die Ziffer niedrig liegt. Die Identifikation bestimmter Mißbildungen des ZNS ist besonders für epidemiologische Studien wichtig. Die Erkenntnis über die multifaktorielle Genese einiger Mißbildungen des ZNS rückt heute immer mehr in den Vordergrund. Von der Ätiologie her gesehen haben der Großteil von Anenzephalie und von Spina bifida wahrscheinlich einen multifaktoriellen Ursprung. Einige, wie z.B. das Meckel-Syndrom oder das Roberts-Syndrom, sind auf grobe Erbstörungen zurückzuführen. Andere, wenn auch seltene Mißbildungen, können mit Chromosomenanomalien gekoppelt sein. Für die präventive Medizin ist es daher besonders wichtig, eine genaue Diagnose zu stellen, um durch genetische Beratung und pränatale Diagnostik weitere Mißbildungen des ZNS verhüten zu können. Dieses Buch setzt sich zum Ziel, dem medizinischen Personal, das sich mit Neugeborenen beschäftigt, eine Nachschlagequelle zu bieten, die es gestatten soll, auf einfache und schnelle Art einige der häufigsten Mißbildungen des ZNS feststellen zu können.

Examination of the newborn infant

Examen du nouveau-né

Untersuchung des Neugeborenen

Examination should be carried out as soon as possible after the birth, but the practice will vary with the circumstances. In some hospitals, paediatricians and specialised nursery staff examine each baby; in others or in domestic circumstances the examination may be undertaken by the midwife or doctor after the mother has been delivered. When there are respiratory problems or the baby is very small, full examination may be delayed until the baby is considered fit to be handled. However, in the recognition of congenital malformations there are some general points which may be helpful as a check list for anyone reading this guide.

General appearance. Observe if the baby is sleeping or awake, pink or blue, and whether or not the limbs move in the appropriate manner. Note any stridor or abnormal cry.

Weight of the baby. The weight should be measured in grams, to the nearest gram, preferably within the first hour of life before significant postnatal weight loss has occurred. 'Low birth weight' is usually defined as less than 2500 g.

Length of the baby. Length may be a useful indicator of the small-for-dates or the baby 'at risk' but may be difficult to measure, especially if the infant is very active.
Crown-heel length is the length from top of head to bottom of the heels when the baby is laid flat, and gently pulled to full extension.
Crown-rump length is the length from top of head to tip of coccyx with the baby lying on its side.

L'examen du nouveau-né doit être effectué aussitôt que possible après la naissance. Dans certaines maternités, tout enfant est examiné par un pédiâtre ou autre spécialiste. Dans d'autres maternités ou lors d'accouchements à domicile, l'examen est pratiqué par la sage-femme ou par le médecin ayant assisté l'accouchement. Lorsque des problèmes respiratoires se posent ou si l'enfant est très prémature, l'examen complet peut être post-posé jusqu'à ce quc l'état de l'enfant le permette. Toutefois, pour poser le diagnostic d'une malformation congénitale, quelques informations générales peuvent être utiles comme liste de vérification.

Aspect général. Observez si le nouveau-né est somnolent ou s'il est éveillé; son teint rosé ou cyanosé; et si les membres se meuvent de façon normale. Remarquez tout stridor ou cri anormal.

Poids de l'enfant. Le poids doit être mesuré en grammes et au gramme près, de préférence endéans la première heure, avant que la perte de poids post-natale ne survienne. Un petit poids de naissance est habituellement défini comme étant inférieur à 2500 g.

Taille de l'enfant. La taille peut être un indicateur utile de dysmaturité mais est parfois difficile à mesurer spécialement si l'enfant est très actif.
La taille sommet du crâne-talons est mesurée, l'enfant couché à plat sur le dos et doucement placé en extension complète.
La taille sommet du crâne-coccyx

Die Untersuchung sollte so bald wie möglich nach der Geburt vorgenommen werden, aber in der Praxis wird es je nach Umständen zu verschiedenen Zeitpunkten erfolgen. In einigen Krankenhäusern untersuchen die Kinderärzte und ein spezialisiertes Plegepersonal jeden Säugling; in anderen Kliniken oder bei Entbindungen zu Hause wird die Hebamme oder der Arzt die Untersuchung sofort nach der Entbindung durchführen. Wenn Atmungsprobleme vorliegen oder der Säugling sehr klein ist; wird die Untersuchung verschoben werden müssen, bis der Säugling kräftiger geworden ist. Nichtsdestoweniger, für die Identifikation von angeborenen Mißbildungen gibt es einige allgemeine Richtlinien, die dem Leser dieses Buches als Anhaltspunkte dienen können.

Allgemeines Aussehen. Beobachten, ob der Säugling schläft oder wach ist, rosig oder blau, und ob die Glieder in natürlicher Weise beweglich sind oder nicht. Auf pfeifendes Atmen oder auf abnormalen Schrei achten.

Körpergewicht. Das Gewicht soll in Gramm und zwar sehr exakt gemessen werden, am besten innerhalb der ersten Stunde nach der Geburt, bevor ein merkbarer postnataler Gewichtsverlust eingetreten ist. Bei einem Gewicht unterhalb 2500 Gramm spricht man von ,niedrigem Geburtsgewicht'.

Körperlänge. Die Körperlänge kann ein nützlicher Faktor sein, um eine fetale Mangelentwicklung (Unreife) des Säuglings festzustellen oder ihn als Risiko-Baby zu

Size of the head. The maximum head circumference is measured by passing the tape round the forehead just above the eyes and round the occiput. Normal measurements for the newborn population should be consulted when deciding whether the head is larger or smaller than normal. A head circumference below second percentile or above the 98th percentile is usually regarded as 'abnormal'.

Shape of the head. Any asymmetry, bulges, or unusual shape of the head should be indicated by a drawing. The presence of any haemangiomas, tufts of hair, or dimples, particularly in the midline, should be noted. The tension and size of the fontanelles should also be documented and the presence of a third fontanelle recorded. Look for the presence of mobile or prominence of cranial sutures.

Limbs. The upper and lower limbs should be examined with special attention to the length between joints, joint shape and joint mobility. The tone of the limbs should be noted particularly if they cannot be straightened or if they are flaccid. The number of fingers and toes, their length, extra digits or fusion of the digits should be noted and any digital abnormality illustrated in a drawing. The presence of abnormal palmar creases must be looked for. Examination for hip dislocation or instability should be undertaken by suitably trained personnel.

Perineum. Inspect the genitalia; in the male note the presence of normal scrotum, penis, foreskin,

est mesurée l'enfant couché sur le côté.

Périmètre crânien. Le périmètre crânien est mesuré en plaçant le mètre ruban autour du front, juste au-dessus des yeux et autour de l'occiput. Une table de référence pour la population locale doit être consultée avant de décider si la circonférence crânienne est supérieure ou inférieure à la normale. Une circonférence inférieure au deuxième percentile ou supérieure au 98ème percentile est considérée comme anormale.

Forme de la tête. Toute assymétrie, bosse ou forme inhabituelle doit être illustrée par un dessin. La présence d'hémangiome, touffe de cheveux ou fossette, particulièrement sur la ligne médiane du crâne, doit être recherchée. La taille et la tension des fontanelles doivent être renseignées, ainsique la présence d'une éventuelle troisième fontanelle. Recherchez également toute suture crânienne mobile ou proéminente.

Membres. Une attention toute particulière doit être apportée à la forme et à la mobilité des articulations des membres supérieurs et inférieurs, ainsi qu'à la longueur entre les articulations. La tonicité des membres doit être vérifiée surtout s'ils ne peuvent être étendus ou s'ils sont flasques. Toute anomalie des doigts ou des orteils, comme anomalie de nombre, de taille, ou fusion, doit être recherchée et reportée par un dessin. La présence éventuelle de plis palmaires anormaux doit être vérifiée. L'examen des hanches en vue du dépistage

bezeichnen. Sie kann aber schwer zu messen sein, besonders wenn der Säugling sehr aktiv bzw. unruhig ist.

Scheitel-Fersen-Länge ist die Länge vom Kopfscheitel bis zum unteren Ende der Fersen, wenn der Säugling flach gelegt und sanft voll ausgestreckt wird.

Scheitel-Steiß-Länge ist die Länge vom Kopfscheitel bis zur Spitze des Steißbeines, wobei der Säugling seitwarts liegt.

Kopfgröße. Den weitesten Kopfumfang mißt man, wenn man das Maß rund um die Stirn legt, knapp über die Augen und um den Hinterkopf herum. Bevor man entscheidet, ob ein Kopf größer oder kleiner als normal ist, soll man die Normalmaße der neugeborenen Bevölkerung in Betracht ziehen. Ein Kopfumfang unter zwei Perzentilen und über achtundneunzig Perzentilen vom Mittelwert wird gewöhnlich als 'abnormal' betrachtet.

Kopfform. Jede Asymmetrie, Beulen oder ungewöhnliche Form des Kopfes soll auf einer Zeichnung vermerkt werden. Das Auftreten von Haemangiomen, Haarbüscheln oder Grübchen, besonders in der Mittellinie, soll vermerkt werden. Die Spannung und Größe der Fontanellen soll auch dokumentiert und das Vorliegen einer dritten Fontanelle registriert werden. Überprüfen, ob bewegliche oder hervorstehende Schädelnähte vorliegen.

Gliedmaßen. Die oberen und unteren Gliedmaßen sollen untersucht und besondere Aufmerksamkeit der Länge

and any abnormal opening in the penis; in the female note the presence of normal labia, and that urinary and vaginal openings are visible and normally situated. Inspect the anus to ensure that it is not imperforate and that there is a normal reflex response to touch.

Skin and hair. Any abnormal texture or discolouring of skin or hair should be described.

Face. The relation of eyes, nose and mouth should be examined, indicating any abnormality with a drawing.

Eyes. The size, shape, and colour of the eyes, any abnormality of the iris and pupil and the presence of a squint or cataracts, should be noted.

Nose. Note the shape, the presence of the septum and whether the nares are patent.

Mouth. Note the size of tongue and any evidence of tongue-tie, and whether roof of mouth complete.

Ears. Observe position and shape, indicating by a diagram relation to head and eyes if their position is abnormal.

Back of the body. Check that the spine is straight and look for any swelling or lump, tuft of hair, haemangiomas or moles overlying the spine. Inspect the shoulders, chest, and pelvis, for symmetry and normal shape.

Front of the body. Note any swellings or asymmetry. Palpate for bladder and renal masses which may

d'une luxation congénitale doit être pratiquée par une personne qualifiée.

Périnée. Examinez les organes génitaux. Chez le garçon, recherchez toute anomalie du scrotum, du penis, du prépuce et du méat urinaire. Chez la fille, recherchez toute anomalie des lèvres du vagin et du méat urinaire. Inspectez l'anus afin de vous assurer qu'il n'y a pas d'imperforation visible et qu'il existe un reflexe normal au toucher.

Peau et cheveux. Toute anomalie de texture ou décoloration de la peau ou des cheveux doit être décrite.

Face. La localisation des yeux, du nez et de la bouche doit être vérifiée et toute anomalie reportée par un dessin.

Yeux. La taille, forme et couleur des yeux, ainsi que toute anomalie de l'iris ou de la pupille, la présence d'un strabisme ou d'une cataracte doivent être notés.

Nez. Observez la forme du nez, la présence de la cloison nasale et vérifiez si les choanes ne sont pas obstruées.

Oreilles. Vérifiez la position et la forme des oreilles et illustrez par un dessin toute anomalie.

Dos. Vérifiez si la colonne vertébrale est droite. Recherchez toute tuméfaction, touffe de poils, hémangiome ou naevus situés sur la colonne. Inspectez la forme des épaules, du thorax et du pelvis afin de repérer une éventuelle asymmétrie.

zwischen den Gelenken gewidmet werden sowie der Form der Gelenke und deren Beweglichkeit. Der Muskeltonus soll überpruft werden, besonders wenn die Gliedmaßen nicht gestreckt werden können oder wenn sie schlaff sind. Die Anzahl der Finger und Zehen, ihre Länge, überzählige Finger und Zehen oder deren Fusion (Verschmelzung) soll festgestellt und jede Anomalie von Fingern und Zehen mit einer Zeichnung illustriert werden. Auf abnormale Falten der Handfläche soll geachtet werden. Eine Prüfung hinsichtlich einer vermutlichen Dislokation oder Labilität des Hüftgelenkes soll von geschultem Personal vorgenommen werden.

Perineum. Geschlechtsorgane überprüfen. Das männliche soll einen normalen Hodensack, den Penis, die Vorhaut aufzeigen. Überprüfen, ob abnormale Öffnungen im Penis vorliegen. Das weibliche Geschlechtsorgan soll normale Labia haben. Die Harn- und Vaginaöffnungen sollen sichtbar und normal situiert sein. Bei Kontrolle des Afters feststellen, ob er nicht durchgängig ist und ob bei Berührung eine normale Reflexantwort vorliegt.

Haut und Haar. Jedes abnormale Gewebe und jede Haut- oder Haarverfärbung soll beschrieben werden.

Gesicht. Das Verhältnis zwischen Augen, Nase und Mund soll überprüft werden und jede Abnormität anhand einer Zeichnung festgehalten werden.

indicate neurogenic bladder or enlarged kidneys.

Biochemical screening. Biochemical tests for phenylketonuria and for congenital hypothyroidism should be carried out at the specific time after birth.

Thorax et abdomen. Notez toute tuméfaction ou asymmétrie. Palpez l'abdomen afin de repérer une éventuelle masse rénale ou vésicale pouvant indiquer une vessie neurogène.

Examens biochimiques. Les examens biochimiques en vue du dépistage de la phénylcétonurie et de l'hypothyroïdie congénitale doivent être effectués en temps voulu après la naissance.

Augen. Größe, Form und Farbe der Augen sollen beachtet werden und jede Abnormität von Iris und Pupille, ein schielender Blick oder grauer Star (Katarakt) angemerkt werden.

Nase. Achten auf die Form, ob die Scheidewand vorhanden ist und die Nasenlöcher durchgängig sind.

Mund. Achten auf die Größe der Zunge, ob Verwachsungen vorliegen und ob das Gaumendach vollständig ist.

Ohren. Achten auf ihre Lage und Form und in ein Diagramm das Verhältnis zum Kopf und zu den Augen zeichnen, insbesondere wenn die Lage der Ohren abnormal ist.

Rücken. Überprüfen, ob das Rückgrat gerade ist; auf jede Geschwulst oder Beule, Haarbüschel, Hämangiome oder Muttermale, die über dem Rückgrat liegen, achten. Überprüfung von Schultern, Brust und Becken, ob sie symmetrisch und normal gebildet sind.

Körpervorderseite. Auf jegliche Geschwulst oder Asymmetrie achten. Durch Betastung von Blase und Nieren überprüfen, ob nicht eine neurogene Harnblase oder vergrößerte Nieren vorliegen.

Biochemische Prüfungen. Biochemische Tests für Phenylketonurie und angeborenen Hypothyreoidismus sollen zu gegebener Zeit durchgeführt werden.

Acephalus

Acéphalie

Azephalus

This disorder is extremely rare and is characterised by total absence of the head.

Cette affection est extrêmement rare et caractérisée par l'absence totale de la tête.

Diese Mißbildung ist außerordentlich selten und wird durch das komplette Fehlen des Kopfes gekennzeichnet.

Anencephalus

Anencéphalie

Anenzephalus

This congenital malformation is characterised by a partial absence of brain tissue and of the cranial vault. The face and eyes are present. Anencephalus may be subdivided into:

Incomplete anencephalus in which the defect does not extend to the level of the foramen magnum (Fig. 1).

Complete anencephalus in which the defect extends through the foramen magnum (Fig. 2).

Craniorachischisis in which complete anencephaly is accompanied by defective closure of the spine (Fig. 3).

Cette malformation congénitale est caractérisée par l'absence partielle du tissu cérébral et de la voûte crânienne. La face et les yeux sont présents. L'anencéphalie peut être subdivisée en:

Anencéphalie incomplète où la malformation ne s'étend pas au-delà du niveau du trou occipital (Fig. 1)

Anencéphalie complète où la malformation s'étend au-delà du niveau du trou occipital (Fig. 2)

Craniorachischisis où l'anencéphalie complète s'accompagne d'un défaut de fermeture de la colonne vertébrale (Fig. 3).

Diese angeborene Mißbildung wird durch das teilweise Fehlen des Hirngewebes und des Schädeldaches gekennzeichnet. Gesicht und Augen sind vorhanden. Der Anenzephalus kann unterteilt werden in:

Unvollständigen Anenzephalus —der Gewebsdefekt erstreckt sich nicht bis zum Hinterhauptsloch (Abb. 1);

Vollständigen Anenzephalus— der Defekt bezieht das Hinterhauptsloch ein (Abb. 2);

Kraniorachischisis—zu dem vollständigen Anenzephalus kommt noch ein mangelhafter Verschluß der Wirbelsäule hinzu (Abb. 3).

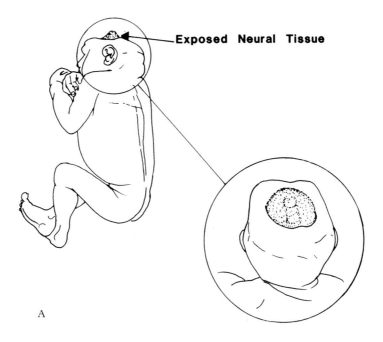

Exposed Neural Tissue

A

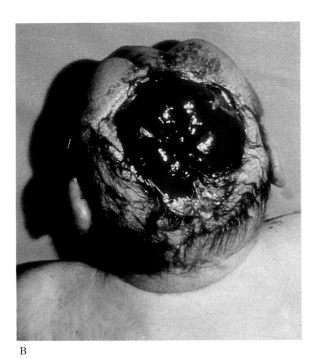

B

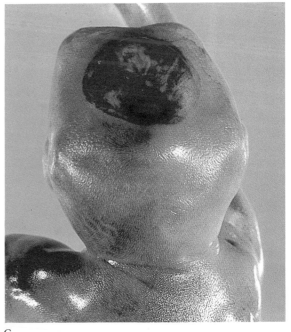

C

Fig. 1 Incomplete anencephalus showing that the defect in the cranial vault does not extend to the level of the foramen magnum.

Fig. 1 Anencéphalie incomplète montrant le défaut de la voûte crânienne ne s'étendant pas au-delà du niveau du trou occipital.

Abb. 1 Unvollständiger Anenzephalus. Der Gewebsdefekt im Schädeldach erreicht nicht das Hinterhauptsloch. Hirngewebe frei liegend.

Exposed   Neural   Tissue

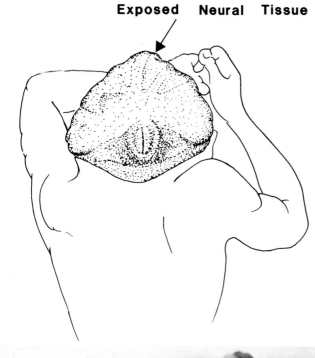

A

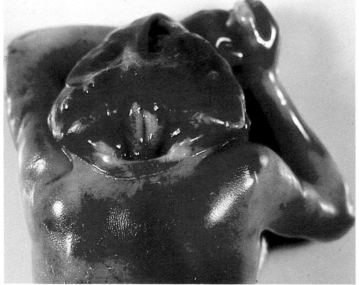

B

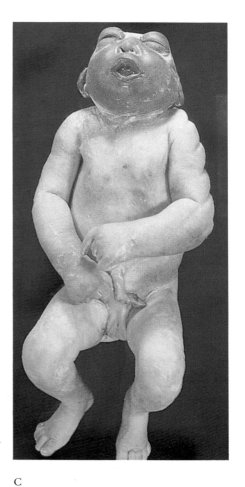

C

Fig. 2 Complete anencephalus illustrating that the cranial defect extends through the foramen magnum. C. shows the typical proptosed eyes and low-set ears.

Fig. 2 Anencéphalie complète illustrant le défaut crânien s'étendant au-delà du niveau du trou occipital. En C, sont indiqués l'aspect typique des yeux et l'implantation basse des oreilles.

Abb. 2 Vollständiger Anenzephalus. Der Schädeldefekt geht durch das Foramen occipitale magnum. C. zeigt die typischen hervorquellenden Augen (Froschaugen) und die tief sitzenden Ohren.

Exposed Neural Tissue

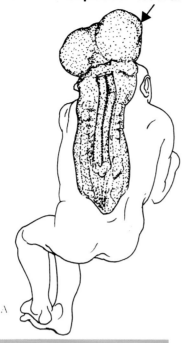

A

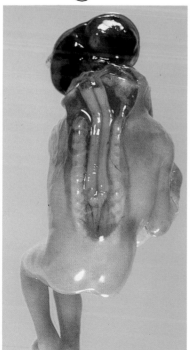

B

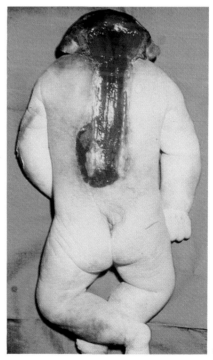

C

Fig. 3 Craniorachischisis in which the complete anencephalus is accompanied by a defective closure of the spine.

Fig. 3 Craniorachischisis où l'anencéphalie complète est associée à un défaut de fermeture de la colonne vertébrale.

Abb. 3 Kraniorachischisis. Der vollständige Anenzephalus wird von einer mangelhaft verschlossenen Wirbelsäule begleitet. Freiliegendes Hirn- und Rückenmarksgewebe.

(Fig. 3C taken from Laurence K.M. 1982. In: Emery A.E.H., Rimoin D.L. (eds). The principles and practice of medical genetics. Churchill Livingstone, Edinburgh, ch. 19. Reproduced with kind permission of the author, editor and publishers.)

Iniencephalus

Iniencéphalie

Inienzephalus

This condition is an anomaly of the foramen magnum and the infant/fetus is characterised by marked retroflexion of the head which is relatively large compared to the trunk. The face looks upwards and there is absence of the neck groove. The skin over the face is continuous with that over the chest and scalp. There may be other associated CNS malformations such as anencephalus (or variants), spina bifida, encephalocele, craniorachischisis, hydrocephalus, or microcephaly (Fig. 4).

Cette affection est caractérisée par une anomalie du trou occipital. L'enfant ou foetus présente une rétroflexion marquée de la tête qui est relativement large par rapport au tronc. La face est dirigée vers le haut et il y a absence du creux cervical. La peau du visage est continue avec celle du thorax et du scalp. D'autres anomalies du SNC comme l'anencéphalie, le spina bifida, l'encéphalocèle, le craniorachischisis, l'hydrocéphalie ou la microcéphalie peuvent y être associées (Fig. 4)

Dieser Zustand entspricht einer Anomalie des Hinterhauptsloches. Der Säugling/Fötus ist dadurch gekennzeichnet, daß der Kopf merklich nach rückwärts gebeugt und verhältnismäßig groß im Vergleich zum Körper ist. Das Gesicht ist nach oben gerichtet und der Hals fehlt völlig. Die Haut geht über Gesicht, Brust und Kopf kontinuierlich über. Es können sich noch andere Mißbildungen des ZNS zugesellen, wie z.B. Anenzephalie oder Varianten, Spina bifida, Enzephalozele, Kraniorachischisis, Hydrozephalus oder Mikrozephalie (Abb. 4).

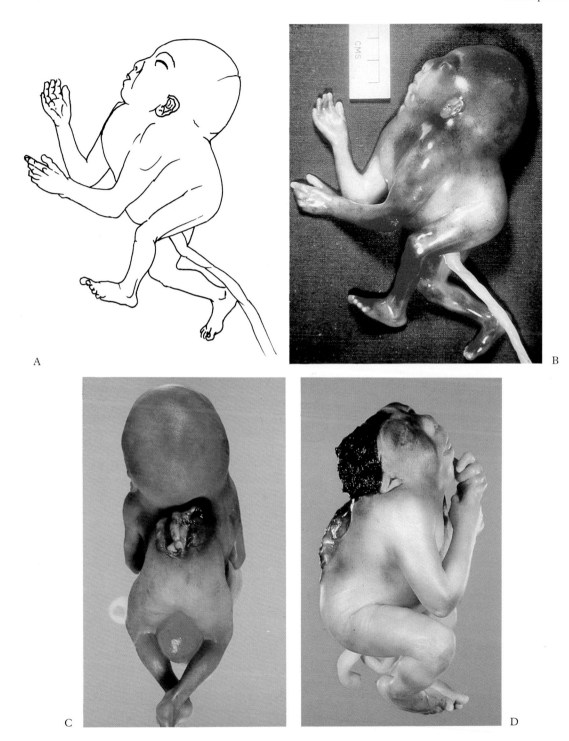

A

B

C

D

Fig. 4 Iniencephalus. A and B show typical appearance with lack of neck groove and upward-looking face. C. shows an associated myelocele. D. shows an associated craniorachischisis.

Fig. 4 Iniencéphalie. A et B montrent une apparence typique avec absence du sillon de la nuque et la face dirigée vers le haut. C montre l'association avec une myélocèle. D montre l'association avec un crâniorachischisis.

Abb. 4 Inienzephalus. A und B. zeigen das typische Erscheinungsbild mit fehlendem Hals und nach oben gerichtetem Gesicht; C. zeigt eine zusätzliche Myelozele; D. eine zusätzliche Kraniorachischisis.

(Fig. 4B taken from Ferguson-Smith M. 1975 Prenatal diagnosis. Ciba Review, Ciba-Geigy, Basle, p. 2. Reproduced with kind permission of the author and publishers.)

Spina bifida

Spina bifida is a midline defect of the osseous spine usually affecting the posterior arches. If the defect is not visible, it is usually described as *spina bifida occulta* of which there are two varieties:

An uncomplicated type in which only one vertebra is affected and there are no associated abnormalities; and

A complicated type in which more than one vertebra is involved with widening of the spinal canal. Externally in the newborn telangiectases, haemangiomas (Fig. 5A), abnormal pigmentation, hypertrichosis (Fig. 5B), lipomas, dimples, dermal sinuses, or dermoid cyst, and in later life, a neurogenic bladder and/or orthopaedic abnormalities, may suggest the underlying osseous defect.

When there is an external protrusion or swelling, the disorder is referred to as *spina bifida cystica* which includes *meningoceles* and *myeloceles*. A meningocele is characterised by a saccular protrusion which involves only meninges (Fig. 6A and B). There is no involvement of the neural elements. The lesion may be covered by normal or atrophic skin. A *myelocele*, however, in addition has involvement of the neural elements (Fig. 6C and Fig. 7A, B, and C). The term myelocele includes myelomeningocele and meningomyelocele.

Spina bifida

Le spina bifida est un défaut de la ligne médiane de la partie osseuse de la colonne vertébrale, affectant habituellement les arches postérieures de celle-ci. Si le défaut n'est pas apparent, il est appelé *spina bifida occulta* dont deux formes sont décrites:

Forme non compliquée où une seule vertèbre est affectée et qui n'est pas associée à d'autres anomalies.

Forme compliquée où plus d'une vertèbre est affectée et qui s'accompagne d'un élargissement du canal rachidien. Extérieurement chez le nouveau-né, des télangiectasies, des hémangiomes (Fig. 5A), une pigmentation anormale de la peau, une hypertrichose (Fig. 5B), un lipome, une fossette, un sinus dermique, un kyste dermoïde ou plus tard, une vessie neurogène et/ou des anomalies orthopédiques peuvent faire suspecter le défaut osseux sous-jascent.

Lorsqu'une protusion est extérieurement présente, l'anomalie est appelée *spina bifida cystica* qui comprend la *méningocèle* et la *myélocèle*. Une *méningocèle* est caractérisée par une protusion sacculaire ne comportant que du tissu méningé (Fig. 6A et B). Il n'y a pas de participation d'éléments nerveux. La lésion peut être couverte de peau normale ou atrophique. Une *myélocèle* implique la présence de tissu nerveux (Fig. 6C et Fig. 7A, B et C). Le terme myélocèle recouvre ceux de myéloméningocèle et méningomyélocèle.

Spina bifida

Die Spina bifida ist ein Mittelliniendefekt der Wirbelsäule und betrifft zumeist die Wirbelbögen. Wenn der Defekt nicht sichtbar ist, bezeichnet man ihn meistens als *Spina bifida occulta*, von der man zwei Varianten kennt:

Ein unkomplizierter Typ, wo nur ein Wirbel befallen ist und keine weiteren Anomalien vorliegen;

Ein komplizierter Typ mit Befall mehrerer Wirbel und Erweiterung des Wirbelkanals. Bei einem Neugeborenen können äußerlich sichtbare Teleangiektasien, Haemangiome (Abb. 5A), Pigmentanomalien, Hypertrichosis (Abb. 5B), Lipome, Grübchen, Hautfisteln (Dermalsinus) oder Dermoidzysten und, im späteren Leben, eine neurogene Harnblase und/oder orthopädische Abnormitäten das Vorliegen von solchen Defekten der Wirbelsäule vermuten lassen.

Wenn eine Schwellung oder eine Geschwulst vorliegt, wird die Fehlbildung als *Spina bifida cystica* bezeichnet, worin *Meningocele* und *Myelozele* inbegriffen sind. Die *Meningozele* ist eine zystenhafte Vorwölbung nur der Hirnhäute (Abb. 6A und B): Nervengewebe ist hier nicht vorhanden. Die Läsion kann von normaler oder atrophischer Haut überzogen sein. Bei einer *Myelozele* dagegen ist im vorgewölbten Sack auch Nervengewebe vorhanden (Abb. 6C und 7A, B und C). Die Bezeichnung Myelozele umfaßt Myelomeningozele und Meningomyelozele.

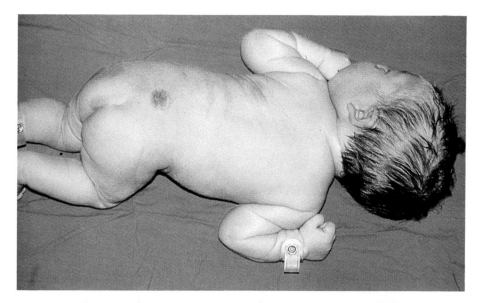

A

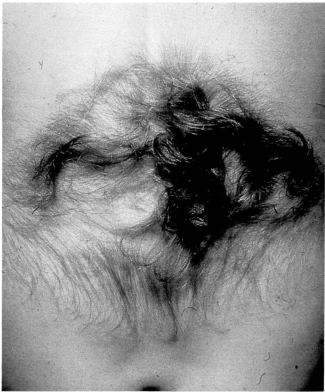

B

Fig. 5 Complicated spina bifida occulta: A. with an associated midline haemangioma in the lumbar region; B. with hypertrichosis in lumbosacral region.

Fig. 5 Spina bifida occulta forme compliquée; A. avec hémangiome médian de la région sacrée; B. avec hypertrichose de la région lombo-sacrée.

Abb. 5 Komplizierte Spina bifida occulta: A. mit einem zusätzlichen Mittellinien-Hämangiom in der Lendengegend; B. mit abnorm starker Behaarung (Hyperthricosis) in der lumbosakralen Gegend.

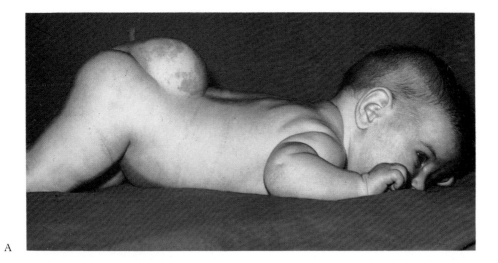

A

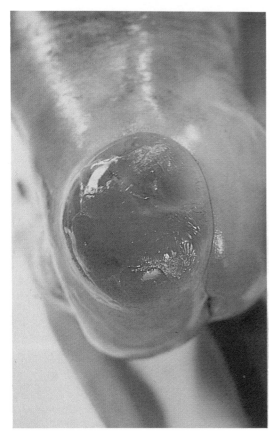

B

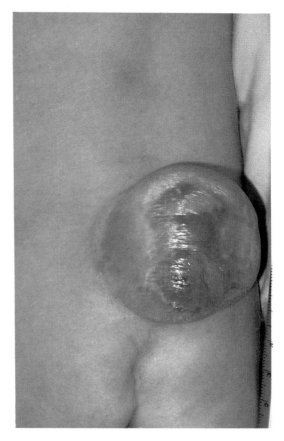

C

Fig. 6 Spina bifida cystica: A. shows a meningocele covered with normal skin; B. a meningocele covered with a thin membrane; C. a myelocele showing involvement of the neural elements.

Fig. 6 Spina bifida cystica; A. Méningocèle couverte de peau saine; B. Méningocèle recouverte d'une fine membrane; C. Myélocèle montrant la participation d'éléments nerveux.

Abb. 6 Spina bifida cystica: A. zeigt eine Meningozele, die mit normaler Haut bedeckt ist; B. eine Meningozele, die von einer dünnen Membran bedeckt ist; C. eine Myelozele mit Einbeziehung von Nervengewebe.

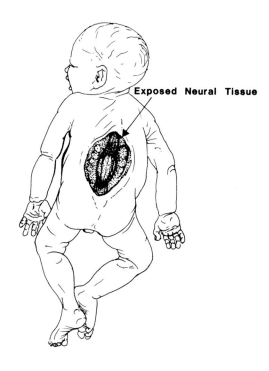

Exposed Neural Tissue

A

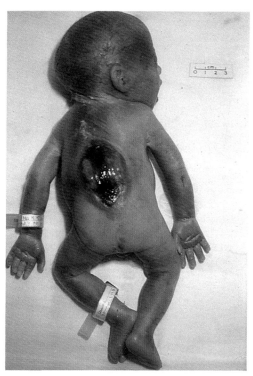

B

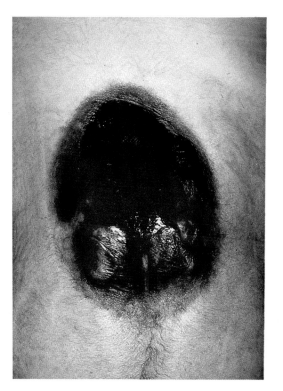

C

Fig. 7 Myelocele with exposed spinal cord.

Fig. 7 Myélocèle avec moëlle épinière exposée.

Abb. 7 Myelozele mit freiliegendem Rückenmark.

Encephalocele

Encéphalocèle

Enzephalozele

This is a cystic expansion of meninges and brain tissue outside the cranium. The lesion may be covered by normal or atrophic skin. The commonest site is in the occipital region (Fig. 8). Occasionally encephaloceles may be frontal, parietal, orbital, nasal or nasopharyngeal.

Il s'agit d'une protusion extracranienne et kystique des méninges et de tissu cérébral. Cette lésion peut être couverte par la peau saine ou atrophique. Le site le plus fréquent de cette lésion est la région occipitale (Fig. 8). Occasionnellement, l'encéphalocèle peut être frontale, parietale, orbitale, nasale ou nasopharyngienne.

Dies ist eine zystische Ausstülpung von Hirnhäuten und Hirngewebe außerhalb des Schädels. Die Läsion kann von normaler oder atrophischer Haut überzogen sein. Am häufigsten tritt sie im Hinterkopf auf (Abb. 8); gelegentlich sind aber die Enzephalozelen auch frontal, parietal, orbital, nasal oder in der Nasen-Rachen-Region vorhanden.

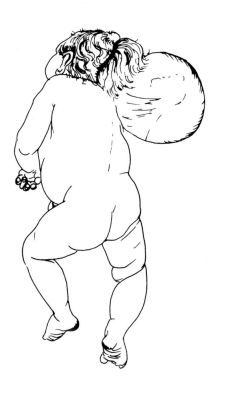

A

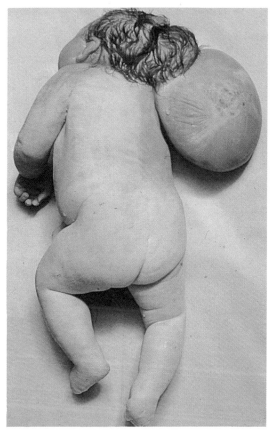

B

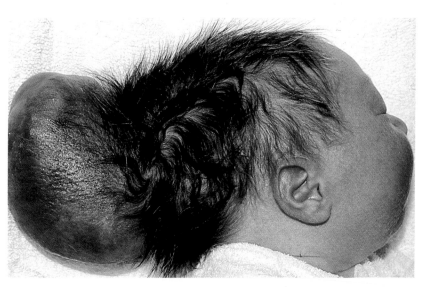

C

Fig. 8 Occipital encephalocele. There is a cystic expansion of the meninges and brain tissue outside the cranium.

Fig. 8 Encéphalocéle occipitale. Il y a expension kystique des méninges et de tissu cérébral en dehors de la voûte crânienne.

Abb. 8 Occipitale Enzephalozele. Extrakranielle zystische Ausstülpung von Hirnhäuten und Hirngewebe.

Cranial meningocele

Méningocèle crânienne

Kraniale Meningozele

This is a cystic expansion of the meninges outside the cranium; it does not contain brain tissue (Fig. 9). The lesion may be covered by normal or atrophic skin.

Il s'agit d'une protusion kystique de tissu méningé en dehors de la voûte crânienne et qui ne contient pas de tissu cérébral (Fig. 9). La lésion peut être recouverte de peau saine ou atrophique.

Dies ist eine zystische Ausstülpung nur der Hirnhäute außerhalb des Schädels, ohne Hirngewebe (Abb. 9). Die Läsion kann von normaler oder atrophischer Haut überzogen sein.

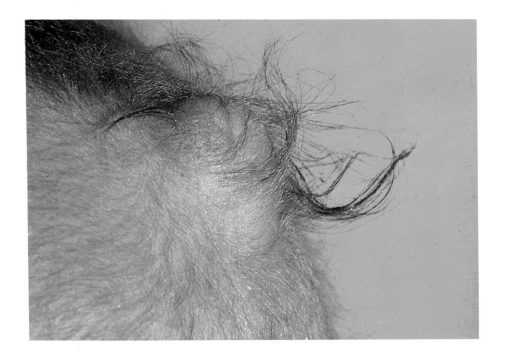

Fig. 9 Cranial meningocele. Cystic expansion of the meninges only. No involvement of brain tissue.

Fig. 9 Méningocèle crânienne. Expansion kystique des méninges sans participation de tissu cérébral.

Abb. 9 Kraniale Meningozele. Zystische Ausstülpung ausschließlich von Hirnhäuten; Hirngewebe ist hier nicht vorhanden.

Cranium bifidum occultum

Cranium bifidum occultum

Cranium bifidum occultum

Focal midline defect in cranium without extrusion of cranial contents, often associated with dermatological abnormalities (Fig. 10).

Défaut médian et focal de la voûte crânienne sans protrusion tissulaire, et souvent associé à des anomalies dermiques (Fig. 10).

Umschriebener Mittelliniendefekt des Schädels ohne Hervorquellen der intrakraniellen Strukturen und häufig mit Hautanomalien verbunden (Abb. 10).

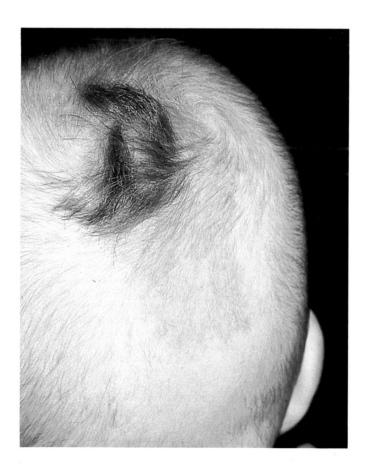

Fig. 10 Cranium bifidum occultum. Localised midline defect with associated haemangioma and darker hair.

Fig. 10 Cranium bifidum occultum. Défaut médian et localisé de la voûte crânienne, associé à un hémangiome et cheveux foncés.

Abb. 10 Cranium bifidum occultum. Umschriebener Mittelliniendefekt mit zusätzlichem Hämangiom und dunklerem Haarbüschel.

Congenital hydrocephalus

Hydrocéphalie congénitale

Angeborener Hydrozephalus (Wasserkopf)

Characterised by dilatation of the ventricular system, not due to primary atrophy of the brain, with or without enlargement of the skull (Fig. 11). Variants include blockage of the aqueduct of Sylvius, blockage of the foramina Magendie and Luscha, blockage of foramen of Monro, and blockage of the basal cistern.

Anomalie caractérisée par une dilatation du système ventriculaire non due à une atrophie primaire du cerveau, avec ou sans élargissement du crâne (Fig. 11). Certaines variétés peuvent être associées à une obstruction de l'aqueduc de Sylvius, du trou de Magendie ou des fentes de Luschka, du trou de Monro ou des citernes basales.

Er ist gekennzeichnet durch eine primäre Erweiterung des Ventrikelsystems, nicht bedingt durch Hirngewebsschwund, mit oder ohne Vergrößerung des Schädels (Abb. 11). Seine Varianten umfassen den Verschluß des Aquaeductus Sylvii oder der Foramina Luschkae und Magendie oder der Foramina Monroi oder die Blockade der basalen Zysternen.

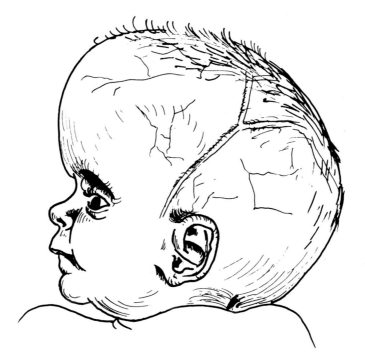

A

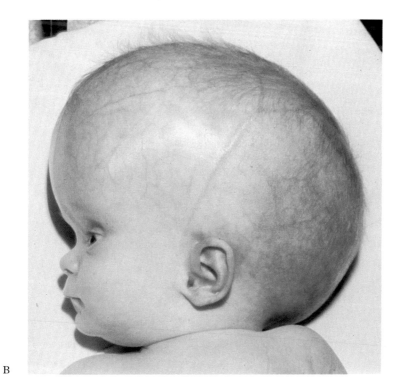

B

Fig. 11 Congenital hydrocephalus showing the generalised enlargement of the head and prominent forehead.

Fig. 11 Hydrocéphalie congénitale montrant l'élargissement généralisé du crâne avec le front proéminent.

Abb. 11 Angeborener Hydrozephalus. Hochgradige Gesamtvergrößerung des Kopfes und vorstehende Stirn.

Arhinencephaly

Arhinencéphalie

Arhinenzephalie

This group of disorders is characterised by an absence of the first cranial (olfactory) nerve tract. There is a spectrum of anomalies from a normal brain, except for the first cranial nerve tract, to a single ventricle (holoprosencephaly). Clinically, there is a spectrum of facies associated with arhincephaly disorders. These include cyclopia (Fig. 12A and B), ethmocephaly (Fig. 12C), cebocephaly (Fig. 13A, B, and C), and hypotelorism with other median facial deformities.

Ce groupe d'anomalies est caractérisé par l'absence de la première paire de nerfs crâniens (nerf olfactif). Toute une gamme d'anomalies cérébrales peuvent être observées, depuis un cerveau normal avec la seule absence du tractus olfactif jusqu'au ventricule unique (holoprosencéphalie). Cliniquement, une série de malformations faciales peuvent être associées à l'arhinencéphalie. Ces malformations faciales incluent la cyclopie (Fig. 12A et B), l'ethmocéphalie (Fig. 12C), la cébocéphalie (Fig. 13A, B et C), et l'hypertélorisme avec d'autres déformations de la face.

Diese Gruppe von Mißbildungen ist gekennzeichnet durch das Fehlen des ersten Hirnnerven bzw. der Riechbahn. Es gibt aber ein ganzes Spektrum von Anomalien: vom normal aussehenden Gehirn mit Fehlen nur der Riechnerven bis hin zur Holoprosenzephalie (mit mißgebildetem Großhirn und einem einzigen Hirnventrikel). Klinisch gesehen gibt es ein weites Spektrum von Gesichtsmißbildungen, die mit Störungen der Arhinenzephalie-Gruppe verbunden sind. Zu ihnen gehören die Zyklopie (Abb. 12A und B), die Ethmozephalie (Abb. 12C), die Zebozephalie (Abb. 13A, B und C) und der Hypotelorismus mit anderen Störungen der Gesichtsmittellinie.

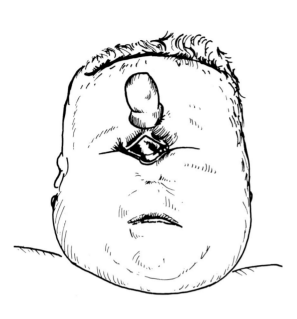

A

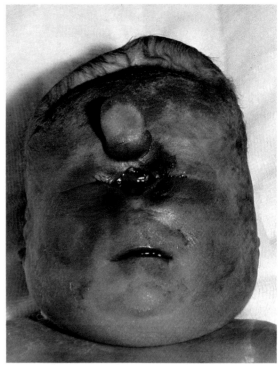

B

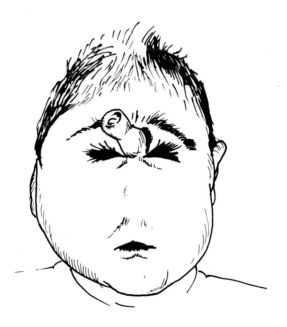

C

Fig. 12 A and B. Typical facies in cyclopia. The proboscis is in the mid-forehead position; C. Ethmocephaly in which the face lacks a nose and the proboscis is attached to the interorbital space.

Fig. 12 A et B. Facies typique de cyclopie. Le proboscis est en position mifrontale; C. Ethmocéphalie avec absence du nez et le proboscis est attaché à l'espace interorbitaire.

Abb. 12 A und B. Typisches Gesichtsbild bei Zyklopie. Die mißgebildete Nase (Rüssel) liegt mitten in der Stirn; C. Ethmozephalie, das Gesicht hat keine Nase, der Rüssel liegt zwischen den Augenhöhlen.

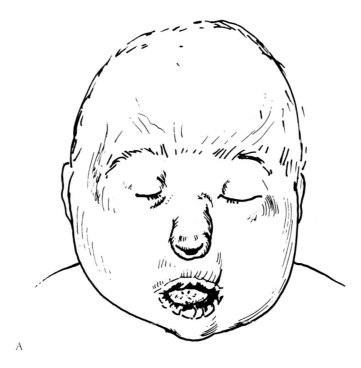

A

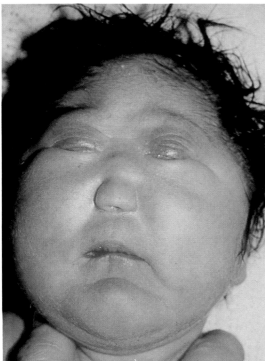

B

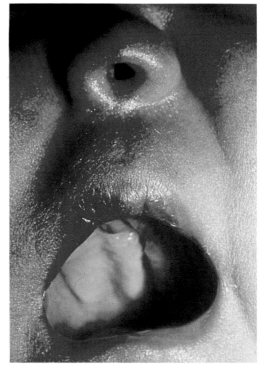

C

Fig. 13 Cebocephaly showing that the orbits have formed and the proboscis has a single nostril.

Fig. 13 Cébocéphalie montrant les orbites formées et le proboscis n'a qu'une narine.

Abb. 13 Zebozephalie. Die Augenhöhlen sind ausgebildet, der Rüssel hat nur ein Nasenloch.

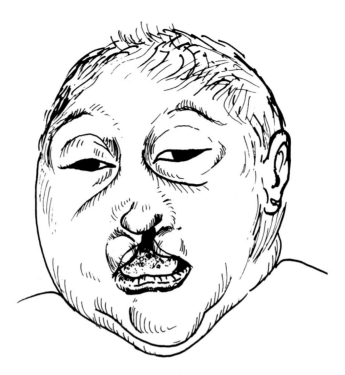

A

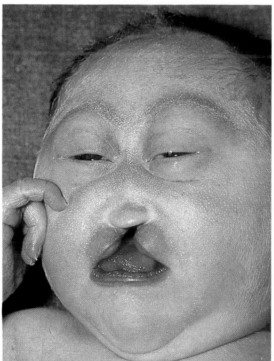

B

Fig. 14 A and B. Orbital hypotelorism with midline cleft lip.

Fig. 14 A et B. Hypertélorisme orbital avec bec de lièvre médian.

Abb. 14 A und B. Orbitaler Hypotelorismus mit medianer Lippenspalte.

Hydranencephaly

Hydranencéphalie

Hydranenzephalie

Bilateral absence of most of cerebral hemispheres particularly the fronto-parietal lobes which are reduced to a translucent membrane enclosing cerebrospinal fluid.

Absence bilatérale de la majeure partie des hémisphères cérébraux, particulièrement des lobes fronto-pariétaux qui sont réduits à une membrane translucide contenant du liquide céphalo-rachidien.

Beiderseitiges Fehlen von Groß-teilen der Gehirnhemisphären, ins-besondere von Stirn- und Schei-tellappen. Sie bestehen oft aus einer dünnen, durchsichtigen Membran, welche die cerebrospinale Flüssig-keit umschließt.

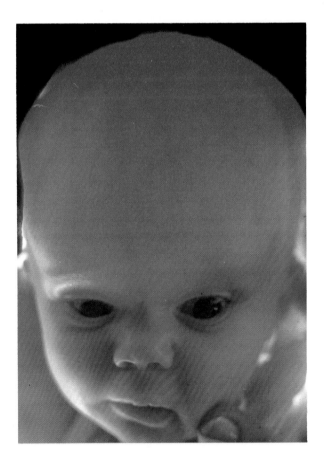

Fig. 15 Hydranencephaly. The skull has been transilluminated to show the replacement of cerebral hemispheres by cerebrospinal fluid.

Fig. 15 Hydranencéphalie. Le crâne a été transilluminé afin de mettre en évidence la présence de liquide céphalo-rachidien en lieu et place des hémisphères cérébraux.

Abb. 15 Hydranenzephalie. Bei Trans-illumination des Schädels sieht man, daß die Großhirnhemisphären nicht vor-handen sind bzw. durch cerebro-spinale Flüssigkeit ersetzt wurden.

Microcephaly

Microcephaly is characterised by a
reduction in the size of the brain
with a skull circumference less than
three standard deviations below the
mean for gestation or age. This may
be associated with a variety of other
anomalies.

Microcéphalie

Cette anomalie est caractérisée par
une réduction de la taille du cerveau
avec réduction de la circonférence
crânienne. Celle-ci est inférieure à
moins de 3 déviations standards par
rapport à la valeur moyenne pour
l'âge. Cette anomalie peut être
associée à une variété d'autres
malformations.

Mikrozephalie

Mikrozephalie ist gekennzeichnet
durch eine Verkleinerung der
Gehirngröße bei Reduktion des
Schädelumfanges um weniger als 3
Normwerte unterhalb der Durch-
schnittswerte der Gestationsperiode
oder des Alters. Diese Mißbildung
kann von einer Vielfalt anderer
Anomalien begleitet werden.

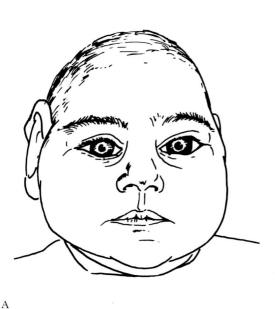

A

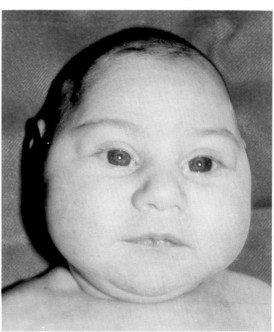

B

Fig. 16 A and B. Microcephaly.　　**Fig. 16** A et B. Microcéphalie.　　**Abb. 16** A und B. Mikrozephalie.

Split notochord syndrome

Malformation neurentérique

Split-Notochord-Syndrom

This syndrome results from a mal-development of vertebral bodies allowing variable contact of neural and visceral elements.

Ce syndrome résulte d'un défaut du développement des corps verté-braux permettant le contact des éléments nerveux et viscéraux.

Dieses Syndrom entsteht durch eine Fehlentwicklung der Wirbelkörper, was in unterschiedlichem Umfang Kontakte von nervösen Strukturen mit den Eingeweiden zur Folge hat.

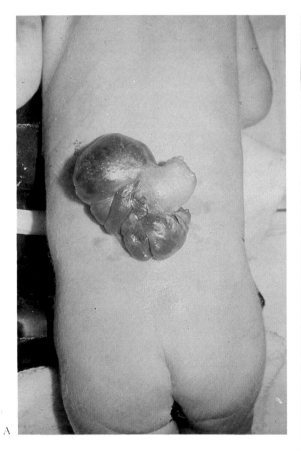
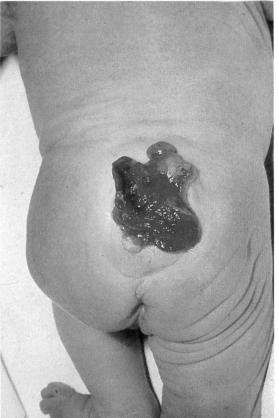

A

B

Fig. 17 Split notochord syndrome showing extrusion of gastro-intestinal tract.

Fig. 17 Malformation neurentérique montrant une protusion externe du tractus intestinal.

Abb. 17 Split-Notochord-Syndrom. Lumbosakrale Prolapse des Magen-Darm-Traktes.

Sacrococcygeal teratoma

Characterised by a swelling of variable size usually situated in the coccygeal region. It is often covered by normal skin but occasionally haemangiomas and ulcers may be observed. Sometimes it may be difficult to distinguish between spina bifida and sacrococcygeal teratoma.

Teratome sacrococcygien

Lésion caractérisée par une tuméfaction de taille variable et habituellement située dans la région sacrococcygienne. Cette tuméfaction est le plus souvent couverte par de la peau saine mais occasionnellement des hémangiomes ou des ulcères peuvent être observés. Parfois, il est difficile de distinguer un teratome sacrococcygien d'un spina bifida.

Saccrococcygeale Teratome

Diese sind Geschwülste von verschiedener Größe, die meistens in der coccygealen Gegend sitzen. Sie sind oft von normaler Haut bedeckt, aber manchmal können sie von Hämangiomen und Geschwüren begleitet werden. Gelegentlich kann es schwer sein, zwischen einer spina bifida und einem saccrococcygealem Teratom zu unterscheiden.

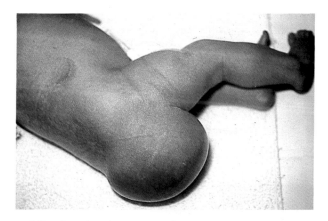

A

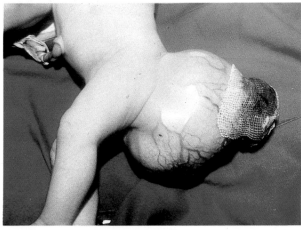

B

Fig. 18 Sacrococcygeal teratoma. A. covered with normal skin; B. showing ulceration.

Fig. 18 Teratome sacrococcygien. A. Couvert de peau saine. B. Montrant les ulcérations.

Abb. 18 Saccrococcygeales Teratom. A. von normaler Haut bedeckt; B. ulzeriert.

Acknowledgements

Remerciements

Danksagungen

We could not have compiled these illustrations of Central Nervous System Malformations without the generous co-operation of colleagues who provided us with slides.

Listed are the individuals who sent us slides: Mr V. Boston, Northern Ireland (Figs. 18A, B), Mr S. Brown, Northern Ireland (Fig. 17A), Mr G. Emerson, Northern Ireland (Figs. 13B, C), Professor M. Ferguson-Smith, Glasgow (Fig. 4B), Dr J. Glasgow, Northern Ireland (Fig. 16B), Mr L.P. Lassman, Newcastle upon Tyne, England (Fig. 17B), Professor K.M. Laurence, Cardiff, Wales (Figs. 3C, 4D, 5B, 15), Professor G. Lyon, Brussels (Fig. 11B), Dr Mastroiacovo, Rome (Fig. 1B). The remaining figures were provided by the Department of Medical Genetics, Northern Ireland. Mr Brendan Ellis, BA, MA (RCA) was responsible for the line drawings. Most of the photography, copying, and reprinting was undertaken by the Department of Photography, Royal Victoria Hospital, Belfast, Northern Ireland. Dr M. Reid, Consultant Neonatologist, Northern Ireland, made several helpful comments concerning the examination of the newborn infant. The authors would like to thank all those persons who have helped with the translation.

L'illustration de ce livre n'aurait pas été possible sans la collaboration des collègues qui ont fourni les documents photographiques originaux.

M. V. Boston, Northern Ireland (Figs 18A, B), M. S. Brown, Northern Ireland (Fig. 17A), M. G. Emerson, Northern Ireland (Figs 13B, C), Professeur M. Ferguson-Smith, Glasgow, Scotland (Fig. 4B), Dr J. Glasgow, Northern Ireland (Fig. 16B), M. L.P. Lassman, Newcastle upon Tyne, England (Fig. 17B), Professeur K.M. Laurence, Cardiff, Wales (Figs 3C, 4D, 5B, 15), Professeur G. Lyon, Bruxelles (Fig. 11B) Dr Mastroiacovo, Rome (Fig. 1B). Les autres illustrations ont été fournies par le Département de Génétique Humaine, Irlande du Nord. M. Brendan Ellis, BA, MA (RCA) est l'auteur des dessins. Le travail de photocomposition a été effectué dans le Département de Photographie du ‹Royal Victoria Hospital›, à Belfast, Irlande du Nord. Le Docteur M. Reid, Consultant Néonatalogiste en Irlande du Nord a apporté ses précieux commentaires pour la partie consacrée à l'examen du nouveau-né. Les auteurs tiennent à remercier les personnes ayant collaboré à la traduction de ce livre.

Ohne die großzügige Hilfe von mehreren Kollegen, die uns Diapositive zur Verfügung gestellt haben, hätten wir dieses Buch von Mißbildungen des Zentralnervensystems nie zusammenstellen können.

Hier ihre Namen: Herr V. Boston, Nordirland (Abb. 18A, B), Herr S. Brown, Nordirland (Abb. 17A), Herr G. Emerson, Nordirland (Abb. 13B, C), Professor M. Ferguson-Smith, Glasgow (Abb. 4B), Dr J. Glasgow, Nordirland (Abb. 16B), Herr L.P. Lassman Newcastle upon Tyne, England (Abb. 17B), Professor K.M. Laurence, Cardiff, Wales (Abb. 3C, 4D, 5B, 15), Professor G. Lyon, Brüssel (Abb. 11B), Dr Mastroiacovo, Rom (Abb. 1B). Alle übrigen Abbildungen stellte das Department of Medical Genetics, Nordirland, zur Verfügung. Herr Brendan Ellis BA, MA (RCA) war für die Zeichnungen verantwortlich. Photographien, Kopien und Reprints wurden hauptsächlich von dem Department of Photography, Royal Victoria Hospital, Belfast, Nordirland, ausgeführt. Dr M. Reid, Consultant für Neonatologie, Nordirland, gab uns viele hilfreiche Anmerkungen zu der Untersuchung des Neugeborenen. Die Autoren möchten allen Leuten danken, denen mit der Übersetzung geholfen haben.

Appendix I

Classification of central nervous system congenital anomalies

Condition	Definition	Variants	Synonyms*
Anencephalus and similar anomalies			
Acephalus	Absence of head		Acrania Acephalic monster Acephalia (Absence of brain) (Agenesis, aplasia of brain)
Anencephalus	Partial absence of brain tissue and of cranial vault; eyes and face present	Incomplete	Hemianencephaly Hemicrania Hemicephaly Meroacrania
		Complete	
		Craniorachischisis	Total dysraphism, (Amyeloencephalus)
Iniencephalus	Anomaly of foramen magnum and cervical vertebrae with retroflexion of head and absence of neck groove	May be associated with anencephaly, spina bifida, microcephaly, hydrocephalus and encephalocele	Closed and open iniencephaly
Spina bifida			
Spina bifida occulta	Only one vertebral arch involved	Uncomplicated	
	More than one arch involved with widening of spinal canal, with or without dermal sinus, lipoma, dermatological or neurological lesion	Complicated	
Spina bifida cystica	Cystic extension of meninges, with or without neural tissue, outside the vertebral canal		Spinal hernia (Imperfect closure) (Hydrocele spinal)
		Meningocele (only meninges)	Hydromeningocele Congenital hernia dura mater
		Myelocele (meninges and neural tissue involved)	Spina bifida aperta (Hydromyelocele), Rachischisis Meningomyelocele, Myelomeningocele Myelocystocele, Myeloschisis
Other congenital anomalies of nervous system			
Cranial meningocele	Cystic expansion of meninges outside the cranium; does not contain brain tissue		Cerebral hernia Imperfect closure skull, Cranium bifidum cystica (pericranial sinus) Cerebral meningocele, (sinus/fistula pericranii)

*See notes at end of table

Appendix I (cont.)

Condition	Definition	Variants	Synonyms*
Encephalocele	Cystic expansion of meninges outside the cranium, containing brain tissue		Hydroencephalocele Hydroencephalomeningocele Cephalocele Encephalomeningocele Encephalomyelocele Congenital hernia brain Congenital hernia of foramina Congenital cerebral hernia Hernia cerebral endaural Meningoencephalocele
Microcephalus	Reduced size of brain with skull circumference less than 3 standard deviations below mean for age	It may be associated with a variety of other brain anomalies	(Hydromicrocephaly), (microencephalon)· (brain hypoplasia), (cephalic hypoplasia) (non-development of brain), (agenesis of skull and skull bones) Microcephaly
Agenesis of corpus callosum	Total or partial absence of the callosal commissure; other parts of the brain being present		Absence, agenesis, hypoplasia or aplasia of corpus callosum
Absence of cerebellum	Varying degrees of hypoplasia		Aplasia, agenesis, reduction deformity, hypoplasia or non-development of cerebellum

Other congenital anomalies of nervous system (cont.)

Condition	Definition	Variants	Synonyms*
Lissencephaly	Unilateral or bilateral reduction or absence of the cerebral convolutions		Agyria Partial or total absence of cerebral gyri Pachygyria Hypoplasia of brain gyri
Micropolygyria	Reduction of the size and increase in number of cerebral gyri		Microgyria Polygyria
Arhinencephaly	Absence of the first cranial (olfactory) nerve and tract	A spectrum of anomalies from normal brain (except for absence of first nerve and tract) to single ventricle (holoprosencephaly)	Alobar holoprosencephaly Cebocephaly, Ethmocephaly Cyclopia Cyclops
Ulegyria	Normal cerebral gyral pattern with atrophic sclerotic gyri		Distortion of gyri Walnut brain

Congenital hydrocephalus

Condition	Definition	Variants	Synonyms*
Congenital hydrocephalus	Dilation of ventricular system not due to primary atrophy of the brain, with or without enlargement of the skull		Communicating or non-communicating internal hydrocephalus, obstructive or non-obstructive hydrocephaly, (congenital macrocephaly)

*See notes at end of table

Appendix I (cont.)

Condition	Definition	Variants	Synonyms[*]
		Blockage of aqueduct of Sylvius	Atresia, anomaly, obstruction, atresia, septum, stenosis, stricture, occlusion of aqueduct with congenital hydrocephalus
		Blockage of foramina of Magendie or Luschka	Blockage foramina 4th ventricle, atresia, obstruction, stricture, occlusion
		Blockage of foramina of Monro	
		Blockage of basal cistern	
		Others	Hypoplasia, imperfect closure of skull or skull bones, absence skull or skull bones, degeneration of brain, distortion of skull or skull bones, anomaly skull or skull bones
		Unspecified	
Hydranencephaly	Bilateral absence of most of cerebral hemispheres. Particularly the fronto-parietal lobes are reduced to a translucent membrane enclosing cerebrospinal fluid		Hydrancephaly (Agenesis of cerebrum)
Arnold-Chiari Malformation	Downward displacement of the cerebellar tonsils through the foramen magnum into the cervical canal, associated with elongation distortion and downward displacement of the medulla oblongata and 4th ventricle		Types I and II Displaced brain Caudal displacement of brain
Dandy Walker Malformation	Cystic dilation of the fourth ventricle with midline cerebellar defect		

Other specified anomalies of brain

Condition	Definition	Variants	Synonyms[*]
Megalencephaly	Pathological hypertrophy of the brain	Hemimegalencephaly	Enlarged brain (Macrocephaly) (Macrogyria)
Porencephaly	Unilateral or bilateral cavities involving the full thickness of the tissue of the cerebral hemisphere		Porencephalic cyst Schizencephaly Single cyst Intracranial congenital cyst
Multiple cerebral cysts	Multiple cysts mainly confined to the white matter and usually not communicating with the ventricular system		Multiple periventricular cysts Leukomalacia Spongy brain (Ectopic cerebrum)
Other specified anomalies of brain			Colloid cyst of third ventricle Heterotopia Malposition Congenital softening (distortion) Progressive degeneration of brain Haematocephalus

[*] See notes at end of table

Appendix I (cont.)

Condition	Definition	Variants	Synonyms*
Other specified anomalies of spinal cord			
Caudal regression syndrome	*Absence of variable length of lower end of spinal cord*		*Atelomyelia*
Diastematomyelia	Duplication of spinal cord always associated with spina bifida		Double or duplication of spinal cord Diplomyelia
Other lesions of cauda equina			Anomaly of cauda equina Defect of cauda equina
Syringomyelia	Cavitation of spinal cord predominantly in upper region		Dilatation of spinal cord Hydromyelia
Split notochord	Maldevelopment of vertebral bodies allowing variable neural and visceral elements		Neurenteric cyst Spinal teratoma
Other specified anomalies			Myelodysplasia Hypoplasia Micromyelia Aplasia, agenesis of spinal cord
Other specified anomalies of nervous system			
Congenital cranial nerve anomalies	Specific nerve involvement, excluding arhinencephaly		Agenesis, aplasia, distortion, atrophy hypoplasia, entrapment by meningeal bands, bone or vessels Nuclear aplasia, of cranial or spinal nerves (mid-position)
Optic nerve			
Acoustic nerve			
Congenital spinal nerve anomaly			
Meninges anomalies (cerebral and spinal)			Congenital adhesions, cysts or malposition of brain tissue Heterotopia cerebralis
Unspecified anomalies of brain, spinal cord & nervous system			
Unspecified anomalies			Distortion, deformity, anomaly malformation (Encephalopathy)

Notes

Riley Day syndrome ⎫
Marcus Gunn syndrome ⎬ Classify these with syndromes or in appropriate organ system
Familial dysautonomia ⎭

* Items in brackets under synonyms are rarely used. It is suggested that these terms should not be used.

Annexe I

Classification des anomalies congenitales du systéme nerveux central

Anomalie	Définition	Variantes	Synonymes*
Anencéphalie et anomalies similaires			
Acéphalie	Absence de la tête		Acephalus (Absence du cerveau) (Agénésie, aplasie cérébrale)
Anencéphalie	Absence partielle du tissu cérébral et de la voûte crânienne; les yeux et la face sont présents	Incomplète Complète Crâniorachischisis	Hémi-anencéphalie, hémicéphalie, hémicrânie Anencephalus, Anencephalomyelie
Iniencéphalie	Anomalie du trou occipital et des vertèbres cervicales avec retroflexion de la tête et absence de la courbure cervicale	Peut-être associé à l'anencéphalie, spina bifida, microcéphalie, hydrocéphalie ou encéphalocèle.	Iniencephalus
Spina bifida			
Spina bifida occulta	Un seul arc vertébral est impliqué	Non-compliqué	
	Plus d'un arc vertébral est impliqué, avec élargissement du canal rachidien, avec ou sans sinus dermique, lipome ou autres lésions dermatologiques ou neurologiques	Compliqué	
Spina bifida cystica	Expansion kystique des méninges en dehors du canal rachidien avec ou sans participation d'éléments nerveux		Spina bifida (Trouble de fermeture du tube neural) (Hydrocèle médullaire) Hydroméningocèle
		Méningocèle (seules méninges)	
		Myélocèle (méninges et éléments nerveux)	Hydromyélocèle, méningomyélocèle, myéloméningocèle, rachischisis, spina bifida aperta, syringomyélocèle, myéloschisis
Autres anomalies du système nerveux			
Meningocèle crânienne	Expansion kystique des méninges en dehors de la voûte crânienne, ne contenant pas de tissu cérébral		(Hydroméningocèle crânienne) (Cranium bifidum cysticum)
Encéphalocèle	Expansion kystique des méninges et de tissu cérébral en dehors de la voûte crânienne		Hydroencéphalocèle Encéphalomyélocèle Encéphaloméningocèle Méningo-encéphalocèle
Microcéphalie	Cerveau de taille réduite avec périmètre crânien inférieur à trois déviations standard sous la moyenne pour l'âge	Peut-être associé à de nombreuses autres anomalies cérébrales	(Hydromicrocéphalie) Microcéphalus Hypoplasie cérébrale Destruction cérébrale, avec réduction de taille du cerveau

*Voyez les notes au fin de la table

Annexe I (cont.)

Anomalie	Définition	Variantes	Synonymes★
Agénésie du corps calleux	Absence partielle ou complète du corps calleux, les autres parties du cerveau étant présentes		Absence, agénésie, hypoplasie, aplasie ou destruction du corps calleux ou de l'ébauche callosale
Absence du cervelet	Divers degrés d'hypoplasie		Aplasie, agénésie, hypoplasie, aplasie du cervelet ou cerebellum
Lissencéphalie	Réduction ou absence unilatérale ou bilatérale des circonvolutions cérébrales		Agyrie Pachygyrie Hypoplaise, absence des circonvolutions cérébrales
Micropolygyrie	Réduction de la taille et augmentation du nombre de circomvolutions cérébrales		Microgyrie Polygyrie
Arhinencéphalie	Absence des bulbes et nerfs olfactifs	Gamme d'anomalies allant de la seule absence des nerfs olfactifs jusqu'au ventricule unique (holoprosencéphalie)	Holoprosencéphalie Cébocéphalie, Ethmocéphalie Cyclopie
Ulegyrie	Atrophie et 'sclérose' de circonvolutions cérébrales dont la disposition topographique est cependant normale		

Hydrocéphalie congénitale

Hydrocéphalie congénitale	Dilatation du système ventriculaire non due à une atrophie primaire du cerveau, avec ou sans élargissement du crâne		(macrocéphalie congénitale) Hydrocéphalie communicante ou non communicante Hydrocéphalie obstructive, hydrocéphalie non-obstructive
		Obstruction de l'aqueduc de Sylvius	Atrésie, sténose, occlusion
		Obstruction du trou de Magendie ou des fentes de Luschka	
		Obstruction du trou de Monro	
		Obstruction des citernes de la base	
		Autres	Disjonction des sutures crâniennes
		Non-spécifié	
Hydranencéphalie	Absence bilatérale de la majeure partie des hémisphères cérébraux. Les lobes fronto-pariétaux sont réduits à une membrane translucide contenant du liquide céphalorachidien		
Malformation d'Arnold-Chiari	Engagement des amygdales cérébelleuses à travers le trou occipital jusque dans le canal rachidien, associé à une élongation et distortion et un déplacement vers le bas du bulbe et du 4ème ventricule		Malformation de Chiari I et II

★Voyez les notes au fin de la table

Annexe I (cont.)

Anomalie	Définition	Variantes	Synonymes*
Malformation de Dandy Walker	Dilatation kystique du 4ème ventricule avec anomalie de la partie médiane du cervelet		
Megalencéphalie	Hypertrophie pathologique du cerveau	Hemimégalencéphalie	(Macrocéphalie) (Macrogyrie)
Porencéphalie	Cavitations unilatérales ou bilatérales entreprenant toute l'épaisseur des hémisphères cérébraux		Kyste porencephalique Kyste congénital intracrânien Schizencéphalie
Kystes cérébraux multiples	Kystes multiples principalement situés dans la substance blanche et ne commuquant habituellement pas avec le système ventriculaire		Kystes périventriculaires multiples Leucomalacie Encéphalomalacie multikystique
Autres anomalies cérébrales			Kyste colloïde du troisième ventricule Hétérotopie Malposition Ramollissement congénital Dégénéressence progressive du cerveau Hematocéphalie

Autres anomalies precisées de la moëlle épinière

Anomalie	Définition	Variantes	Synonymes*
Syndrome de régression caudale	Absence d'une portion variable de l'extrémité inférieure de la moëlle épinière		Atelomyelie
Diastematomyelie	Duplication de la moëlle épinière toujours associée à un spina bifida		Diplomyelie Duplication de la moëlle épinière Moëlle double

Autres lesions de la queue de cheval

Anomalie	Définition	Variantes	Synonymes*
Syringomyelie	Cavitation de la moëlle épinière principalement de sa portion supérieure		Hydromyélie Dilatation de la moëlle épinière
Malformations neurenteriques	Anomalie du développement des corps vertébraux conduisant au contact entre des éléments nerveux et viscéraux		Kyste neurentérique Teratome rachidien Kystes spinaux entérogènes
Autres anomalies			Myélodysplasie Hypoplasie medullaire Micromyélie Aplasie, agénésie de la moëlle épinière

Autres anomalies precisées du système nerveux

Anomalie	Définition	Variantes	Synonymes*
Anomalie congénitale des nerfs crâniens	Anomalie spécifique de nerfs crâniens, excluant l'arhinencéphalie		Agénésie, aplasie, distortion, atrophie, hypoplasie, compression de nerfs crâniens Aplasie nucléaire des nerfs crâniens ou rachidiens

*Voyez les notes au fin de la table

Annexe I (cont.)

Anomalie	Définition	Variantes	Synonymes*
Nerf optique			
Nerf acoustique			
Nerf rachidien			
Meninges (cerebrales et medullaires)			Hétérotopie cérébrale Adhérences, kystes, malposition

Anomalies du cerveau, moëlle épinière et système nerveux, sans precision

Anomalies, sans precision			Distortion, déformation, anomalie, malformation (Encéphalopathie)

Remarque:

Syndrome de Riley Day
Syndrome de Marcus Gunn   } Ces syndromes doivent être classés dans la partie réservée aux syndromes ou dans le système anatomique
Dysautonomie familiale   approprié

*Les termes entre parenthèses sont rarement utilisés. On suggére que ces termes ne soient pas utilisés.

Anhang I

Klassifikation der angeborenen Anomalien des zentralen Nervensystems

Zustand	Definition	Varianten	Synonyma*
Anenzephalus und ähnliche Anomalien			
Azephalus	Fehlen des Kopfes		Akranie Azephales Monstrum Azephalie (Fehlen des Gehirns) (Agenesie, Aplasie des Gehirns)
Anenzephalus	Partielles Fehlen von Hirngewebe und Schädeldach; Augen und Gesicht vorhanden	Unvollständig Vollständig Kraniorachischisis	Hemianenzephalie Hemikranie Hemizephalie Meroakranie Totaler Dysraphismus (Amyeloenzephalus)
Inienzephalus	Rückwärtsstellung des Kopfes, fehlender Hals	Kann auftreten zusammen mit Anenzephalie, Spina bifida, Microzephalie Hydrozephalus und Enzephalozele	Verschlossen oder offen Inienzephalie
Spina bifida			
Spina bifida occulta	Nur ein Wirbelbogen ist betroffen	Unkompliziert	
	Mehrere Wirbelbögen sind betroffen mit Erweiterung des Wirbelkanals, mit oder ohne Hautfisteln, Lipome, dermatologische oder neurologische Läsionen	Kompliziert	
Spina bifida cystica	Zystische Ausstülpung der Hirnhäute, mit oder ohne Nervengewebe, ausserhalb der Wirbelsäule		Spinale Hernie (Unvollkommener Verschluss) (Spinale Hydrozele)
		Meningozele (nur Meningen) Myelozele (enthält Meningen und Nervengewebe)	Hydromeningozele Angeborene Hernia Durae matris—Spina bifida aperta, (Hydromyelozele) Rachischisis Meningomyelozele Myelomeningozele Myelozystozele Myeloschisis

*s. Anmerkungen am Ende der Tabellen

Anhang I (Fortsetzung)

Zustand	Definition	Varianten	Synonyma*
Angeborener Hydrozephalus			
Angeborener Hydrozephalus	Erweiterung der Hirnventrikel, nicht durch Hirnatrophie entstanden, mit oder ohne Vergrößerung des Schädels		Kommunizierender oder nicht kommunizierender interner Hydrozephalus obstruktiver oder nicht obstruktiver Hydrozephalus (Angeborene Makrozephalie)
		Blockade des Aquaeductus Sylvii	Atresie, Anomalie Obstruktion Atresia, Septum Stenosis, Striktur, Aquäduktverschluß mit angeborenem Hydrozephalus
		Verschluß der Foramina Magendie oder Luschkae	Blockade der Foramina des 4ten Ventrikels Atresie, Striktur Okklusion
		Verschluß der Foramina Monroi	
		Verschluß der basalen Zisterne	
		Andere	Hypoplasie. Unvollständiger Verschluss des Schädels oder der Schädelknochen, Fehlen des Schädels oder der Schädel-
		Nicht spezifiziert	knochen, Degeneration des Gehirns, Distorsion des Schädels oder der Schädelknochen, Anomalie des Schädels oder der Schädelknochen
Hydranenzephalie	Beiderseitiges Fehlen großer Teile der Großhirnhemisphären Besonders die Stirn- und Scheitellappen sind zu einer dünnen, durchsichtigen, die cerebro-spinale Flüssigkeit umschließende Membran reduziert		Hydranzephalie (Agenesis des Zerebrums)
Arnold-Chiari Missbildung	Verlagerung der Kleinhirnton-sillen nach unten durch das Foramen Magnum in den Zer-vikalkanal, begleitet von einer Distorsion-Verlängerung und caudaler Verschiebung der Medulla oblongata und des 4ten Ventrikels		Typen I und II Verschobenes Gehirn Caudale Verschiebung des Gehirns
Dandy Walker Missbildung	Zystische Erweiterung des vierten Ventrikels mit Defekt des Kleinhirnwurmes		
Andere spezifische Anomalien des Gehirns			
Megalenzephalie	Pathologische Hypertrophie des Gehirns	Hemimegalenzephalie	Gehirnvergrösserung (Makrozephalie) (Makrogyria)

*s. Anmerkungen am Ende der Tabellen

Anhang I (Fortsetzung)

Zustand	Definition	Varianten	Synonyma*
Porenzephalie	Einseitige oder beiderseitige Hohlräume in den Großhirnhemisphären, die gesamte Gewebedicke betreffend		Porenzephalische Zyste Schizenzephalie Einzelzyste Intrakranielle angeborene Zyste
Multiple zerebrale Zysten	Mehrfache Zysten, meistens des Marklagers, und gewöhnlich nicht mit dem Ventrikelsystem kommunizierend		Multiple periventriculare Zysten Leukomalacien Schwammiges Gehirn (Ectopisches Zerebrum)
Andere spezifische Anomalien des Gehirns			Kolloidzyste des dritten Ventrikels Heterotopie Fehllage Angeborene Erweichung (Distorsion) Progressive Degeneration des Gehirns Haematozephalus

Andere angeborene Anomalien des Nervensystems

Zustand	Definition	Varianten	Synonyma*
Kraniale Meningozele	Zystische Ausstülpung der Hirnhäute ausserhalb des Schädels; enthält kein Hirngewebe		Zerebrale Hernie Unvollkommener Schädelverschluss Cranium bifidum cysticum (Perikranieller Sinus)
Enzephalozele	Zystische Ausstülpung der Hirnhäute ausserhalb des Schädels, Hirngewebe enthaltend		Zerebrale Meningozele, (Sinus/fistula pericranii) Hydroenzephalozele Hydroenzephalomeningozele Zephalozele Enzephalomeningozele Enzephalomyelozele Angeborene Gehirn Hernie Angeborene Foramina-Hernie Angeborene zerebrale Hernie Hernia cerebral endaural Meningoenzephalozele
Mikrozephalus	Reduzierte Grösse des Gehirns mit Schädelumfang unterhalb 3 Standardwerte von den mittleren Normwerten für das Alter	Kann von verschiedenen anderen Hirnanomalien begleitet werden	(Hydromicrozephalie) (Microencephalon) (Gehirnhypoplasie) (Mangelentwicklung des Gehirns) (Agenesis von Schädel und Schädelknochen) Mikrozephalie
Agenesie des Corpus callosum	Vollständiges oder unvollständiges Fehlen des Balkens andere Teile des Gehirns sind vorhanden		Fehlen, Agenesie Hypoplasie oder Aplasie des Corpus callosum

*s. Anmerkungen am Ende der Tabellen

Anhang I (Fortsetzung)

Zustand	Definition	Varianten	Synonyma*
Fehlen des Cerebellum	Verschiedene Stufen von Hypoplasie		Aplasie, Agenesie Reduktionsdeformität, Hypoplasie oder Nichtentwicklung des Cerebellum
Lissenzephalie	Einseitige oder beiderseitige Reduktion oder Fehlen der Gehirnwindungen		Agyrie partielles oder komplettes Fehlen der zerebralen Gyri Pachygyria Hypoplasie der Gehirnwindungen
Mikropolygyrie	Abnahme der Grösse und Zunahme der Anzahl der Gehirnwindungen		Mikrogyrie Polygyrie
Arhinenzephalie	Fehlen der ersten Hirnnerven und Bahnen (Riechhirn)	Ein Spektrum von Anomalien vom normalen Gehirn (abgesehen vom Fehlen des N. olfactorius) bis hin zum monoventrikulären Hirn (Holoprosencephalie)	Alobar Holoprosenzephalie Zebozephalie Ethmozephalie Zyklopie Cyclops
Ulegyrie	Normales Muster der Gehirnwindungen mit atrophisch sklerotischen Windungen		Distorsion der Gyri Wallnusshirn

Andere spezifische Anomalien des Rückenmarks

Zustand	Definition	Varianten	Synonyma*
Caudales Regressions Syndrom	Fehlen oder unterschiedliche Länge des unteren Endes des Rückenmarks		Atelomyelia
Diastematomyelia	Rückenmarks-Verdoppelung, immer begleitet von Spina bifida		Verdopplung des Rückenmarks Diplomyelia
Andere Veranderungen der Cauda equina			Anomalie der Cauda equina Defekt der Cauda equina
Syringomyelia	Aushöhlung des Rückenmarks, vorwiegend der oberen Abschnitte		Rückenmarkserweiterung Hydromyelia
Split-Notochord	Fehlentwicklung der Wirbelkörper mit Zusammentreffen in unterschiedlichem Ausmaß von nervösen Strukturen und Eingeweide		Neurenterische Zyste Spinales Teratom
Andere spezifische Anomalien			Myelodisplasie Hypoplasie Micromyelie Aplasie Agenesie des Rückenmarks

*s. Anmerkungen am Ende der Tabellen

Anhang I (Fortsetzung)

Zustand	Definition	Varianten	Synonyma*
Andere spezifische Anomalien des Nervensystems			
Angeborene Kranial-nerven Anomalien	Spezifische Nervenveränderungen, ausgeschlossen Arhinencephalie		Agenesie, Aplasie Distorsion, Atrophie Hypoplasie Veränderungen durch Meningealstränge Knochen oder Blutgefässe Nukleare Aplasie der kranialen oder spinalen Nerven (Mediale Position)
Sehnerv			
Hörnerv			
Angeborene Anomalie der Spinalnerven			
Hirnhäute-Anomalien kranial oder spinal			Angeborene Verwachsungen, Zysten oder Fehllage des Gehirngewebes Heterotopia cerebralis
Nicht spezifizierte Anomalien von Gehirn, Rückenmark und Nervensystem			
Nicht spezifizierte Anomalien			Distorsion, Deformität, anomale Mißbildung (Enzephalopatie)

Anmerkungen

Riley Day Syndrom
Marcus Gunn Syndrom   } Diese sind unter Syndromen oder dem zugehörigen organischen System einzureihen
Familiäre Dysautonomie

*Die Benennungen in Klammern unter den Synonyma werden selten verwendet. Es wird empfohlen, diese Bezeichnungen nicht mehr anzuwenden.

Appendix II

Annexe II

Anhang II

List of EUROCAT centres*

Liste des centres EUROCAT*

Liste der EUROCAT-Zentren*

Name of register Nom du registre Referenzzentrum	Country Pays Land	Register leader Directeur Leiter	Address Adresse Adresse
Hainaut	Belgium	Dr I. Borlee	Ecole de Santé Publique UCL-EPID 30.34 Clos Chapelle-aux-Champs 30 B–1200 Bruxelles Tel: (02) 762.34.00 Ext: 3325
W. Vlaanderen	Belgium	Prof. R. Beckers	Ministerie Van Volksgezonheid en van het Gezin Administratief Centrum Vesaliusgebouw B–1010 Brussel Tel: (02) 564.80.11 prive: (050) 33.21.82
Odense	Denmark	Dr M. Ulrich	University of Odense Dept. of Clinical Genetics 17, J.B. Winslowsvej DK–5000 Odense C Tel: (09) 12.71.79
Berlin	Germany	Dr G. Karkut	Dept. Gynae. and Obstetrics Free University Berlin 45 Hindenburgdamm 30 Tel: (030) 798.25.93
Evia	Greece	Dr S. Tsagaraki	Children's Hospital Agia Sophia Institut of Child Health GR–Athens 617 Tel: Athens 7708291
Firenze	Italy	Dr C. Galanti	Assessorato Della Sanita Dipartimento Sicurezza Sociale 26 Via di Novoli I–Firenze CAP 50100 Tel: (055) 27.661
Roma	Italy	Dr P. Mastroiacovo	Istituto di Pediatria University Cattolica Largo Agostino Gemelli 8 I–00168 Roma Tel: Rome 33051
Emilia Romagna	Italy	Dr E. Calzolari	Istituto di Genetica Medica I–Ferrara Italy Tel:

*1982

List of EUROCAT centres*		Liste des centres EUROCAT*	Liste der EUROCAT-Zentren*
Name of register *Nom du registre* *Referenzzentrum*	*Country* *Pays* *Land*	*Register leader* *Directeur* *Leiter*	*Address* *Adresse* *Adresse*
Strasbourg	France	Dr C. Stoll	Départment de Medécine Génétique University de Strasbourg F. Strasbourg (Bas Rhin)
Paris-Yvelines	France	Dr (Mme) J. Goujard	Groupe de Recherches Epidémiologique sur la Mère et l'Enfant INSERM 44 Chemin de Ronde F–78110 Le Vésinet Tel: Paris 976 3333
Dublin	Ireland	Dr Radic	The Medico-Social Research Board 73 Lower Baggot Street IRL–Dublin 2 Tel: (01) 76.11.76 (01) 76.60.76
Galway	Ireland	Dr D.F. Lillis	Regional Hospital IRL, Galway Tel: (91) 64141
Luxembourg	Luxembourg	Dr D. Hansen-Koenig	Ministère de la Santé Publique Division de Médecine Préventive et Sociale 10 av. de la Liberté L–Luxembourg Tel: 40801
Groningen	The Netherlands	Dr L.P. ten Kate	Dept. of Human Genetics University of Groningen 4, A. Deusinglaan NL–Groningen
Glasgow	United Kingdom	Dr F. Hamilton	Greater Glasgow Health Board 351 Sauchiehall Street GB–Glasgow G2 3HT Tel: (041) 332.29.77
Liverpool	United Kingdom	Prof. F. Harris	Institute of Child Health Dept. of Child Health Alder Hey Children's Hospital Eaton Road GB–Liverpool L12 2AP Tel: (051) 228 2024
Belfast	United Kingdom	Prof. N.C. Nevin	The Queen's University of Belfast Dept. of Medical Genetics Institute of Clinical Science Grosvenor Road GB–Belfast BT12 6BJ Tel: 40.503 ext: 392

Cataloguing data

British Library Cataloguing in Publication Data
Nevin, Norman C.
    Illustrated guide to malformations of the central
nervous system at birth.
    1. Central nervous system—Abnormalities
    2. Infants (Newborn)
    I. Title   II. Weatherall, Josephine A.C.
    III. Commission of the European Communities
    616.8′0443   RC362

CIP-Kurztitelaufnahme der Deutschen Bibliothek
Nevin, Norman C.:
Illustrated guide to malformations of the central
nervous system at birth = Illustrierter Leitfaden
der Missbildungen des Zentralnervensystems bei der
Geburt/Norman C. Nevin; Josephine A. C.
Weatherall. Comm. of the European Communities.—
Stuttgart: Enke, 1983.
NE: Weatherall, Josephine A. C.:

Library of Congress Cataloging in Publication Data
Nevin, Norman Cummings.
    Illustrated guide to malformations of the
central nervous system at birth.
    Added t.p.'s in French and German.
    'Produced as one of the outcomes of a work-
shop on the recording of central nervous
system malformations held in Brussels in
December 1979 as part of the EUROCAT co-
ordination program.'
    1. Central nervous system—Abnormalities—
Diagnosis. 2. Pediatric neurology—Diagnosis.
3. Infants (Newborn)—Medical examinations.
I. Weatherall, Josephine Alice Coreen.
II. Title. [DNLM: 1. Central nervous system—
Abnormalities—Congresses. 2. Abnormalities—
Diagnosis—Congresses. WL 300 R311 1979]
RJ290.N48 618.92′80443   82-1224
                AACR2

ISBN 0 443 02635 1 (Churchill Livingstone)
ISBN 3 432 93191 3 (Enke)